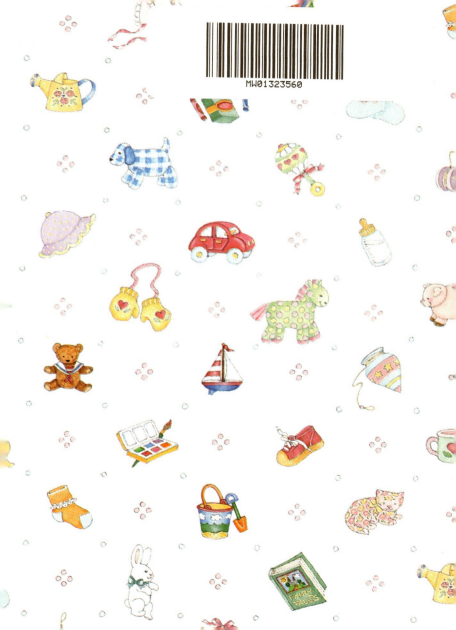

July 4, 1995

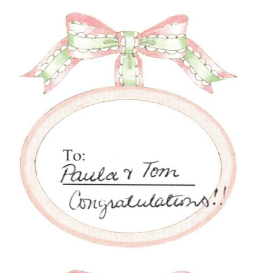

To:
Paula & Tom
Congratulations!!

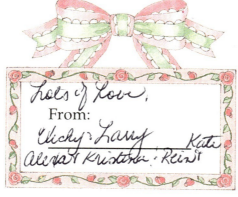

Lots of Love,
From:
Vicky & Larry
Alexa & Kristina & Reini, Kati

Text Copyright © MCMXCIII Jane Parker Resnick
Art Copyright © MCMLXXXIX by Mothers' Aid of Chicago Lying-in Hospital
All rights reserved.
No part of this book may be reproduced in any form or by any means,
electronic or mechanical, including photocopying,
recording, or by any information storage and retrieval system
without the written permission of the publisher.
Published by The C.R. Gibson Company, Norwalk, Connecticut 06856
ISBN 0-8378-5299-4
GB665

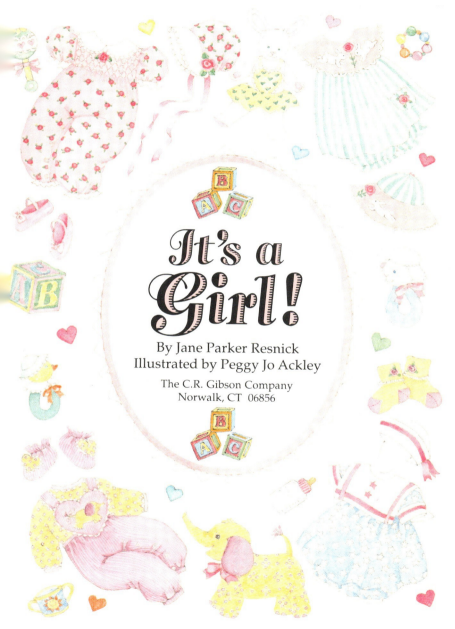

It's a Girl!

By Jane Parker Resnick
Illustrated by Peggy Jo Ackley

The C.R. Gibson Company
Norwalk, CT 06856

A little girl is yours today and nothing will ever be the same. Her life is new and yours is too, for every day will bring some change. For this moment, hold her close and watch her sleep. Feel the joy that fills your heart. Let time stand still and enjoy the miracle of your beautiful baby girl.

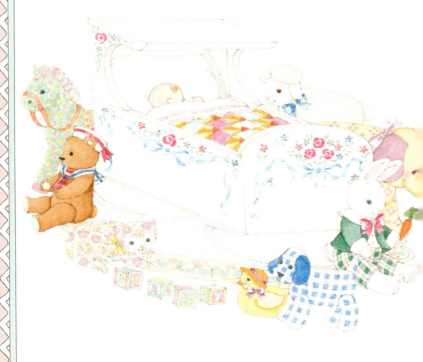

Your baby girl's so helpless and small.
She's not at all the girl she's going to be.
Not ready for playing house or dancing school…
Not ready for figuring out the rules
Of what's allowed and what is not.
Her every need is in your hands,
You strive to meet each new demand.
She'll grow and change, your love will, too.
Now is just the beginning.
There's so much to look forward to.

Your baby needs just two things to make her grow.

Food to feed her body and love to nourish her soul. And when you respond to these demands she'll receive something else—yourself.

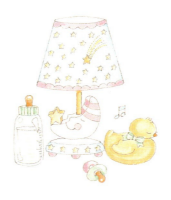

*Sometimes it seems
This child of your dreams
Was born to keep you up at night,
And make each meal a hectic fright.
But even when she cries to let you know
That she intends to keep you on the go,
You still won't think that she's a pest.
For she's your baby, not like the rest,
You know that you are truly blessed.*

For nine months this baby girl was safe and warm within her mother's body. Now she is separate. Hold her in your arms and keep her safe and wrap her in your love to keep her warm. And then she'll know, no matter where she is, she'll never be alone.

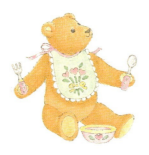

Babies do seem to come with a great deal of paraphernalia. A whole family embarking on a camping trip seems to have less equipment than this tiny baby girl. A crib is a necessity—everyone needs a place to sleep. But then . . . the changing table and diaper pail, the playpen and swing, the high chair and car seat, the walker and stroller. . . and that's the first year. What's to come?

More, of course, plus a long list of things just for fun.

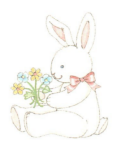

*You can tell your baby "I love you,"
But she won't understand the words,
The love you express
Comes through your hands,
Your smile, your arms
And the sweet sound of your voice.
Hold her and touch her
As if she were a flower,
Delicate and beautiful,
Yet filled with a power
That makes you love her in every way,
From the very first moment,
Of the very first day.*

If the sweetness of your baby girl could be captured as perfume, you could hold it for the future to enjoy in years to come. But those baby smiles are fleeting and those infant yawns are brief. So place them in your memory to cherish them again.

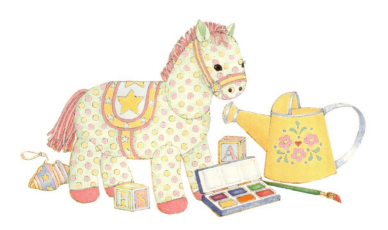

*Growing and changing
Is what babies do best
One day this precious child
May behave like all the rest.*

Someday she'll close her door and ask that a knock be given for permission to enter a place that looks as if a clothes convention were being held on the floor. She'll talk on the phone and roll her eyes with a sigh that says, "It's my parents." Girls are like that somewhere in between being a baby and a young lady. Remember, that time does pass. Slowly.

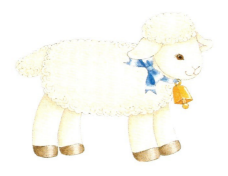

It won't be long before your girl has a "baby" doll of her own—bedraggled, pulled out of shape, missing parts, but irreplaceable. The doll goes where she goes, sleeps where she sleeps and is never far from sight. If you watch carefully you will see that the love your little girl lavishes on this doll is the love she learned from you. Take heart—you've given her a good start.

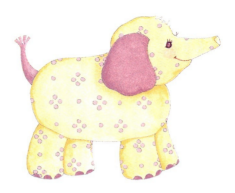

Pretty soon your baby girl will reach for the world. Carry her on your shoulders and she'll grab—the person standing near, the dish on the shelf, the curtain rod—your ear. Most of what she wants you'll have to refuse.

Except for you—and that's all she really needs.

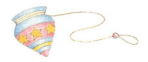

There's something new in the house.
Even the silence
Is filled with excitement.
Every hush is just a time
In-between when the baby cries.
For when your baby girl is up
The world's a newborn place,
Full of wonder
Drenched with love.
A home filled with joy
By a little girl's grace.

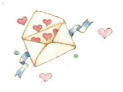

Your baby knows you by your touch, for her eyes can barely see. So the beauty of holding her is more than just the pleasure of her baby softness. Your caress and her infant grasp are the language of a newborn love.

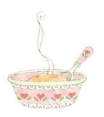

With the birth of this child, there's gladness that never existed before and happiness newly defined. Who would have thought that a tiny baby girl could bring such surprising delight?

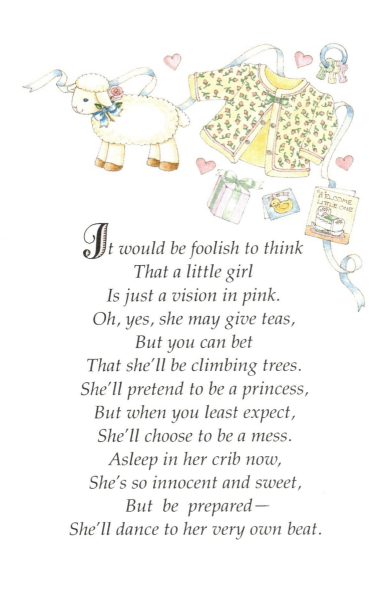

*It would be foolish to think
That a little girl
Is just a vision in pink.
Oh, yes, she may give teas,
But you can bet
That she'll be climbing trees.
She'll pretend to be a princess,
But when you least expect,
She'll choose to be a mess.
Asleep in her crib now,
She's so innocent and sweet,
But be prepared—
She'll dance to her very own beat.*

There can never be too much gentleness for a baby girl.

The tenderness you show her is what she'll come to expect. Through your affection, she'll learn what she needs to know—that gentleness and tenderness are gifts that she can give, too.

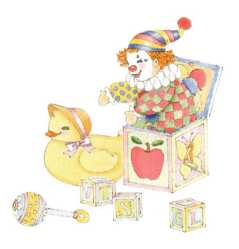

Play "pat-a-cake" with your baby girl and give her a ride on your knees. Throw her in the air and catch her. Sing a silly song. Because giggles count and laughter matters and humor is more than fun. Show her that there's joy in life and you want it to be hers.

*Baby girls have a way of charming
That's completely disarming.
They counter all objections
With cute protestations
Until we gladly give in
No matter what their sin.
And you'll be no different
With this tiny infant.
For she'll steal all your days,
With her sweet, baby ways.*

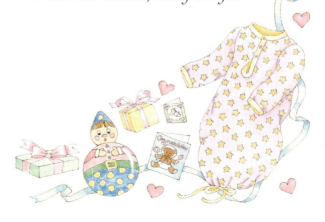

Remember this: The first time your baby girl smiles you are seeing the twinkle of a newborn fire.

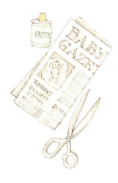

Lucky child to have parents who will cherish her as if the world depended on her existence. Because your world does. Lucky parents to have a girl to treasure you with a love that will light your lives.

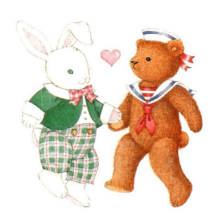

The intensity of the love you feel for this baby girl is so powerful. For the moment, everything else recedes.

Life as you knew it before is merely background. Life as it will be is barely imagined. For now, today and this baby girl are all that matter.

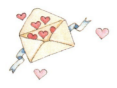

*Whoever said girls were born to please
Has probably never heard "no"
Uttered in the voice of a stubborn young lady;
Has probably never seen the steel
In the eyes of a beauty queen;
Sugar and spice and everything nice
Are not, for girls, the only combination.
Expect a girl with a mind of her own.
Imagine what this infant will become,
A wonder, a surprising joy to behold.*

This baby girl has come to you as a package without directions. A newborn without clues. But the bond between you is a thread of exquisite awareness. Intuitively, you will guess what she needs. Instinctively, you will know what she wants. With this connection, love provides the directions.

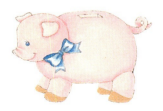

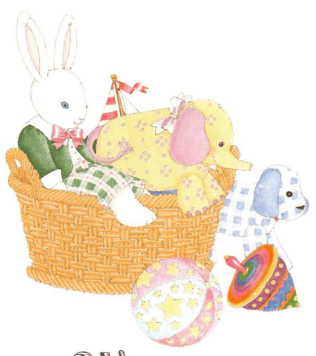

*Watch her explore
her tiny universe—
and then outgrow it.
She moves on,
expands her horizons,
broadens her view—
and yours, too.*

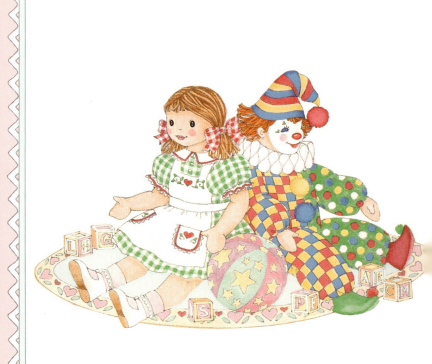

You have been born into a new life. You step, with new understanding, into your place on the family tree. Open your heart with gratitude for this gift from your newborn child.

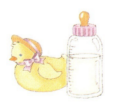

Sleepless nights, busy days—a haze of baby cries and sighs. You'll never be at a loss for something to do, for with a baby there's always something new. Seeing the world from her point of view, you'll never be bored. She's ready for anything. Are you?

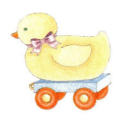

You've had a baby — you're in for a treat.
With a girl, life will always be sweet.
She'll bring a softness to your days,
And happy moments with her gentle ways.
She'll fill the house with little girl toys,
Dolls and dishes and chattering noise.
With hugs and kisses right from the start,
She'll win you over and melt your heart.

*We will try to be good parents,
but we know that love alone
is not enough.
Help us turn love into teaching,
shape love into guidance.
Lead her toward that special light
so that she may be kind,
generous, and loving;
show our daughter the joy of life
so she may grow toward happiness.*

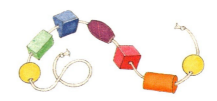

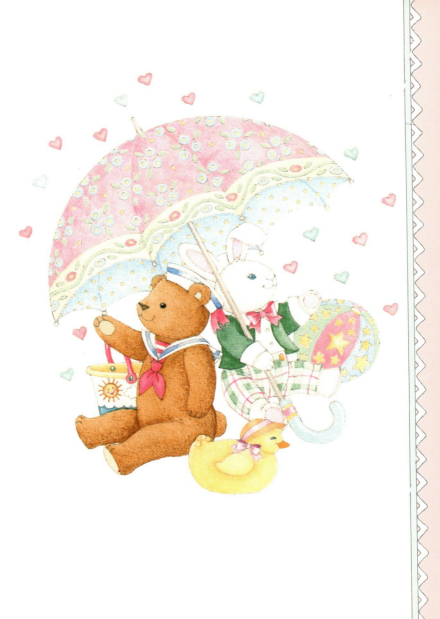

Colophon

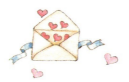

Graphic Designer: Aurora C. Lyman

Typeset in Palatino, Palatino Italic and Garrick

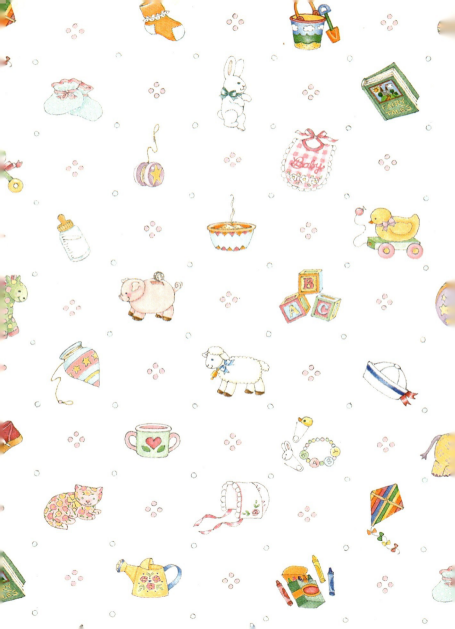